Contents

Introduction

What thoughts crowd your mind when considering starting a singing for health choir? Hurdles to overcome? Singers becoming ill during sessions and looking to you for help? Both are possible and highly likely at some point. Even at this early stage you may sense the degree of preparation and commitment required, yet also how rewarding and fulfilling this could be for you and your participants and, crucially, that your efforts have the potential to change lives. A singing for health (SfH) choir becomes a family for many and a lifeline to some. So proceed with enthusiasm: it's worth it.

What's the difference?

Do SfH choirs differ from regular singing groups? Experienced choir facilitators will be familiar with the challenge of group management, the politics of interpersonal relationships and the potentially emotive nature of repertoire choice. In this respect SfH choirs are indistinguishable from ordinary choirs. Yet in other ways their unique purpose poses challenges that require particular consideration. This guide aims to provide tips and practical advice regarding session management, preparation of mind and body and choice of repertoire. It is aimed at anyone interested in running a group, but particularly those with less formal musical experience who realise the potential benefits of singing and seek a helping hand to get started.

Who attends a SfH choir?

Singing for health choirs historically exist for participants with specific conditions including mental health issues, COPD (a respiratory disease), Parkinson's and Alzheimer's disease. Commonly, however, the outlook is holistic rather than specific and participants who do not have a diagnosed condition are equally keen to attend, appreciating the activity of singing as beneficial to their general health and wellbeing. Friends, family and carers are usually encouraged to take part since the activity of singing together can be an effective equaliser within carer-dependent relationships, encouraging shared participation and fulfilment.

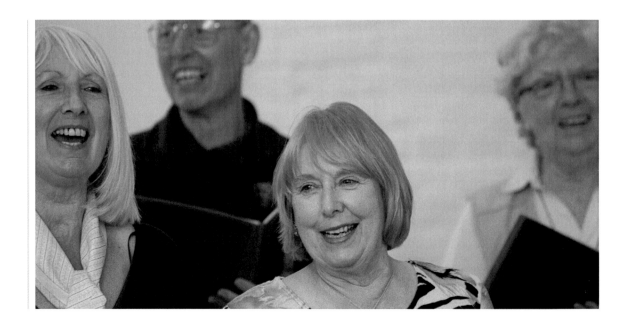

Sidney De Haan
Research Centre for Arts and Health

Singing for Health: Tips and Tactics
A practical guide to running a singing for health choir

Series Editor: Stephen Clift

The aim of this series is to offer guidance on setting up and running singing groups for people with a range of enduring health issues.

They are based on previous research, the learning from singing for health projects in the UK, and the practical experience of members of the Sidney De Haan Research Centre in establishing and evaluating community singing projects since 2004.

1. Singing and Mental Health – Ian Morrison and Stephen Clift

2. Singing and people with COPD – Ian Morrison and Stephen Clift

3. Singing and people with Dementia – Trish Vella-Burrows

4. Singing and people with Parkinson's – Trish Vella-Burrows and Grenville Hancox

5. Singing for Health: Tips and Tactics – Sonia Page

Further resources to supplement this guide can be found online at:
www.canterbury.ac.uk/research/centres/SDHR

For further information on training courses associated with these resources please contact Isobel Salisbury, Sidney De Haan Research Centre for Arts and Health, Canterbury Christ Church University, 65-69 The Block, Tontine Street, Folkestone, Kent, England, CT20 1JR   Email: Isobel.Salisbury@canterbury.ac.uk   Telephone: 01303 220 870

The Sidney De Haan Research Centre for Arts and Health would like to thank everyone who helped with the development of this guide: Julia Baldwin-Jones, Phoene Cave, Chris Price, Matthew Shipton, Kathy Stewart, Trish Vella-Burrows and Pauline Waugh.

Author: Sonia Page   Publisher: Canterbury Christ Church University
Published: February 2014   ISBN: 9781909067066

Sidney De Haan
Research Centre for Arts and Health

A practical guide to running
a singing for health choir

Singing for Health: Tips and Tactics

Sonia Page

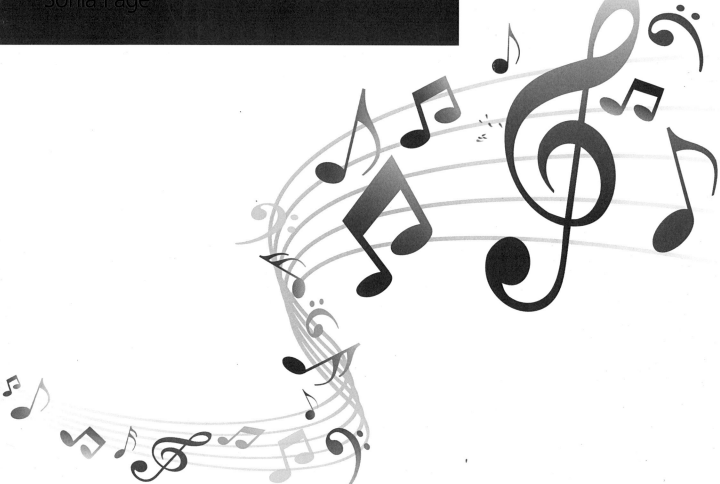

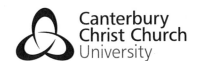
Canterbury
Christ Church
University

Wails of the unexpected

Serious problems are, mercifully, few and far between and this section does not address management of medical emergencies or acute social problems. If a participant appears unwell enough to require medical attention always call an ambulance (or appropriate emergency help if meeting in a medical institution). The reality is that you probably can't do very much to assist other than reassure and get help. It may be useful to have contact details to hand for Social Services or local support groups to give to individuals in times of difficulty.

What follows is a selection of potential scenarios with suggested solutions, none of which is prescriptive but may serve as a guide.

'We don't like the songs you've chosen!'

The curse of choir leadership and responsible for many hours of nocturnal wakefulness.
Consider the following:

- Who chooses the material?
- Are you solely responsible or do participants make suggestions?
- Do you take on board their suggestions?
- Are the majority happy?
- What specific health benefits are you aiming for, for example, increased breath control?

It is often impossible to please everyone and the group should respect your decisions. Equally you may find it helpful to allow suggestions but this can be problematic as inappropriate choices do more harm than good. A variety of leadership models exist ranging from authoritarian to partnership in style. Whichever you adopt, be flexible but decisive; if the majority are happy then the repertoire is fine.

'The songs are too high/low'

Check the range of your material carefully. Untrained older voices may find singing a higher range challenging and should not be strained – see Warm-ups: preparing and protecting the voice. Individuals may not know whether they are soprano or alto (female), tenor or bass (male). Occasionally you may find a male alto but these individuals generally know they are such and have a formal singing history. More likely you will find ladies who think they are tenors. Genuine female tenors are rare but some ladies are more comfortable singing with the men.

- It is advisable to start with songs spanning a mid-range, for example A below middle C to C above middle C.

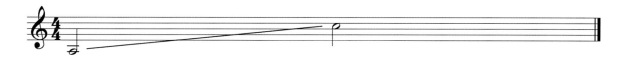

- Choose your starting note for each song prior to the session
- Practise yourself; if it feels too high or low then it probably is
- CHECK: are participants employing good posture and breathing techniques? If not they will struggle whatever the range.

'I can't get my breath while singing'

Some participants may have physical conditions that affect their breathing and it may not be obvious to you, the facilitator. It is normal for novice singers to experience some degree of breathlessness, but this should improve over subsequent sessions.

Tips for avoiding problems include:

- CHECK: are participants employing good posture and breathing techniques? If not they will struggle to get a good initial inhalation and supported exhalation

- Are you starting the song clearly to allow a full, initial inspiration?

- Allow participants to breathe as required when singing a new song

- To encourage a more polished performance, identify phrases that might be sung in one breath but keep them short. A uniform breathing pattern when singing can enhance a choir's performance and is not reliant upon long phrases

- Participants with asthma or COPD may benefit from taking their reliever inhaler prior to the session

- If a participant experiences breathing difficulties during a session make sure they stop singing, sit down and use a reliever inhaler if they have one. Do not assume they are asthmatic; get emergency help if they do not recover speedily

Don't panic! It is uncommon for participants to experience significant breathing difficulties caused by singing and you should not be afraid to encourage phrasing and performance. No one will collapse because of your direction and they will take a breath if it is required.

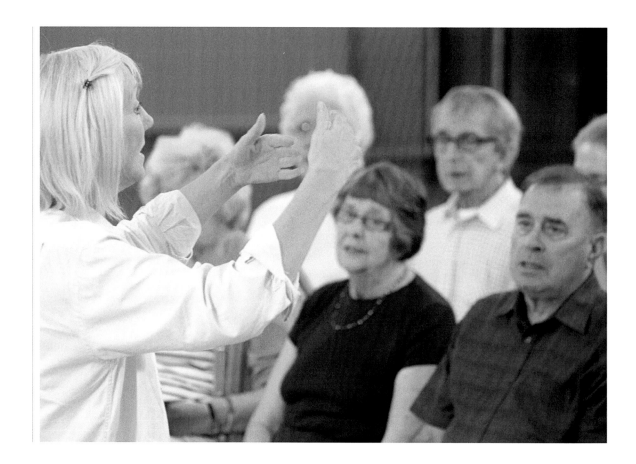

Warm-ups

Why warm-up?

The importance of a warm-up routine cannot be overstated. Effective warm-up exercises prepare both mind and body for singing and, vitally, help to protect the vocal cords from damage. Do not assume that amateur singers need to prepare any less than professionals.

You may find the process of warming up also assists with the following:

- Defines the start of the session and settles the group prior to singing
- Focuses participants' attention on the facilitator
- Encourages a neutral atmosphere on which the facilitator may build the session
- Promotes commonality within the group

When to warm-up?

Always start a session with warm-ups. You may find it useful to 'reset' the group at a mid-way point by revisiting some of the physical warm-up exercises. Often this technique is used to ensure correct posture and remind participants of the need to think about breathing technique and voice production throughout the session. If appropriate, it may be useful to end the session with relaxed breathing exercises.

What types of warm-up should I include?

Ideally both physical and vocal warm ups, as well as opportunity to relax the mind, focus on breath-control and sound production (see examples in Vocal exercises).

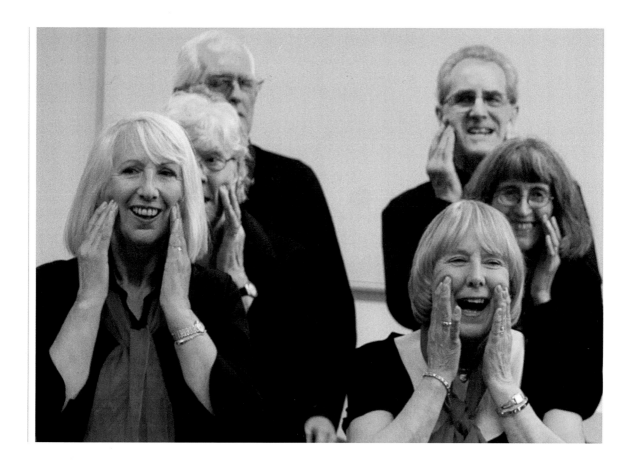

Preparing mind and body to sing

These examples of physical and vocal warm-up exercises are not prescriptive. Each facilitator will have their own ideas and should be encouraged to develop an individual style of delivery, as well as innovative variants. Singing groups catering for members with a variety of long-term conditions have successfully used the following routine.

Posture

- Stand up straight or sit up if unable to stand
- If standing, ensure weight evenly spread between both legs
- Relax knees and loosen shoulders
- Ensure head is straight, tilting neither to the side nor up or down
- Close your eyes and concentrate on yourself
- Adopt a relaxed smile
- Open your eyes

Think of this position as being in 'neutral'. It may be useful to refer to this during the session and encourage participants to return to 'neutral' which should quickly reset any slumped posture or physical tension.

Head and face

- Turn head slowly from side to side; return to neutral
- Raise head gently to look at the ceiling; return to neutral
- Give a gentle yawn; repeat with a relaxed smile and raised eyebrows
- Open mouth wider with a yawn and relax open
- Keeping lower jaw loose, wiggle it gently from side to side
- Chew an imaginary toffee; repeat with mouth open
- Try to keep that 'just-yawned' feeling in the mouth, i.e. raised soft palate and open throat

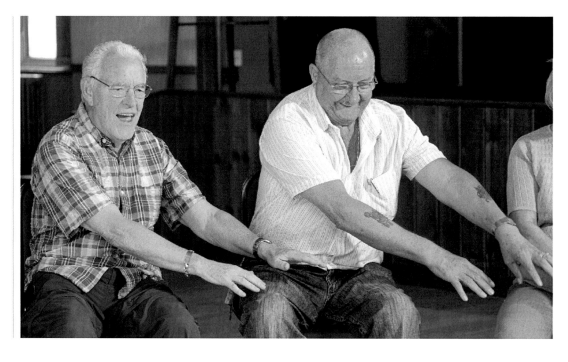

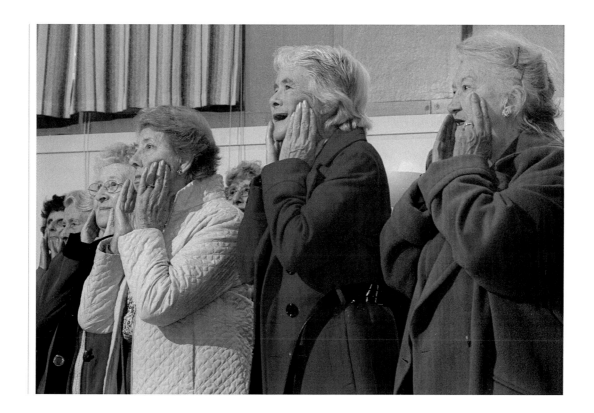

Upper and lower body

- Roll shoulders backward and forward to loosen muscles
- Raise arms high above the head and wave at the ceiling
- Lower arms and wave at the floor
- Swing arms independently ('spaghetti arms') while gently twisting torso
- March on the spot, or lift one leg then another if unable to stand
- If able, lift one foot at a time and rotate it gently

The emphasis should be on relaxed, controlled movements. Encourage your group to multitask by combining different exercises. For example, marching on the spot while performing 'spaghetti arms' and smiling stimulates brain and body as well as promoting laughter, itself a fine precursor to singing.

Breathing

The challenge for facilitators is to encourage participants to take control of their breathing rather than being at the mercy of it. This is especially relevant for those with respiratory or heart disease – and some may have both – which cause varying degrees of breathlessness both at rest and upon exertion. Some participants will be used to functioning while rarely taking a deep breath and the fear of breathlessness can be a powerful and negative influence on daily activities. The facilitator has the opportunity here to empower and positively affect every part of a participant's life by encouraging simple, but effective, breath control. The importance of these or any similar breathing exercises cannot be overstated.

> Remember: it is entirely normal for those who are new to singing to find themselves slightly breathless. Your participants will know their limits and will not over-exert themselves.

The act of breathing

This exercise focuses the mind on the act of breathing and effectively calms and prepares the group to work on their breath control.

- Maintaining a relaxed physical posture, take slow, deep breaths in and out
  Note: inhaling through the nose warms the air and reduces upper airway irritation, coughing and discomfort. Exhale through the mouth.

- Imagine you are filling up deep into your abdomen; do not tighten your waist; keep shoulders down and soft when breathing in

- Breathe in, then very gently and inaudibly, exhale fully

- CHECK: discourage shoulder lifting during the act of breathing

The breathing cycle

Over a period of time the breathing cycle encourages the singer to extend their exhalation while remaining in control. As well as building respiratory muscle strength it is a great confidence-booster for those who struggle with breathlessness.

- Exhale fully

- Inhale while relaxing the abdominal muscles; feel as though the abdomen is filling with air

- Inhale still further; fill up the middle of your chest; note how the rib cage expands

- Hold your breath for a moment

- Exhale as gently and slowly as possible; as air is expelled pull your abdominal muscles in to force out remaining breath

- Let everything go

- Now repeat the breathing cycle but increase the exhalation to a slow count of 6

- A starting speed of 1 count per second may be appropriate.

- Gradually increase the exhalation length to 8, 10 and 12 etc. as group is able*.

*Note: it may take some weeks to achieve this.

It is useful to repeat the breathing cycle at least once during the singing session to remind participants of the need to think about their breathing. It may be a good time to check general posture and readjust as necessary.

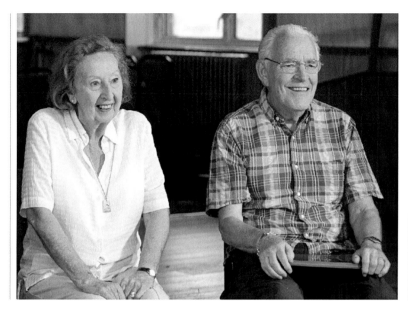
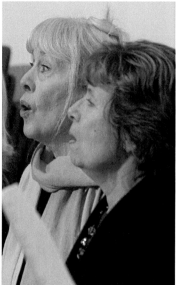

Preparing and protecting the voice

It is worth reminding participants that their vocal cords are ligaments activated by tiny muscles that respond to exercise. Older vocal cords may have lost strength and bulk, and while there is every reason to sing and give them a workout this should be undertaken gently. The idea is to gradually improve over time and enjoy regular, effective singing.

Certain medications and inhalers may cause a dry, irritable throat. In addition, some participants may have vocal nodules or other irregularities that affect their ability to sing comfortably - and they will ask you, the facilitator, what to do about it.

Basic Rules

- Hydrate the vocal cords by drinking plenty of water throughout each day
- Avoid smoking and second-hand smoke where possible
- Do not strain the voice - gently does it
- Relax! Participants may become tense immediately prior to singing
- Practise: encourage participants to practise the breathing exercises and to sing between sessions to promote flexible, toned vocal cords
- Participants who are aware of vocal cord irregularities should seek medical advice prior to singing
- If participants complain of pain in their throat when singing recheck their posture, breathing and state of relaxation. If pain persists stop singing and advise them to seek a medical opinion.

Facilitators should encourage a gentle, easy tone that avoids harsh or strained singing. A light, soft tone supported by the diaphragm will strengthen over time without straining the apparatus, allowing the natural singing voice to develop.

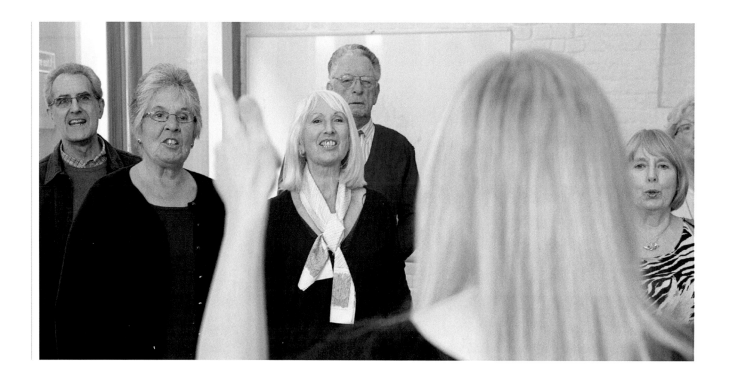

Vocal exercises

The following vocal exercises progress the participant through breath control to sound production and into singing. They are an example of material currently used by singing for health groups and you should be encouraged to develop your own ideas and material to provide variety.

Tip: remind participants of posture and a relaxed smile; the tendency is to tense up and frown once singing commences.

Laughing

- Start with gentle laughter moving through upper and lower range
- Repeat laughter supporting from diaphragm rather than a 'throaty' tone

Humming on 'N'

- Inhale deeply then gently hum on a mid-range note to the letter 'N'
- Repeat starting on 'N' and progress to 'NYAH'; ensure open mouths and relaxed posture; move slowly from 'N' through 'Y' into the vowel sound
- Repeat on ascending and descending scale but neither too high nor low

Sirens

- Siren swoops: starting mid-range, mimic a siren swooping first up then down; try this on different vowel sounds.
- Repeat the siren swoops while 'blowing a raspberry' - requires strong diaphragmatic control to sustain the sound and is great fun!

Counting exercise

- Inhale; while exhaling sing the numbers 1-10 very softly on one note as many times as possible in one breath
- Repeat; concentrate on releasing as little air as possible to avoid a breathy tone
- Remember the purpose of warm-up exercises is to prepare the voice, not to wear it out at the start of the session.
- Participants may try to over-sing the warm-ups; encourage a gentle tone and continually readjust posture and breathing.
- Once again: encourage participants to maintain a good posture and employ the breathing techniques throughout the session. The tendency is to 'slump' the minute warm-ups are finished and 'proper singing' begins.

Tip: be clear and concise when counting the beat and especially at the start of the exercise. Participants will learn quickly if you demonstrate as well as describe.

Fizz and blow

This fizz and blow exercise encourages full inhalation and develops control of exhalation.

Sonia Page

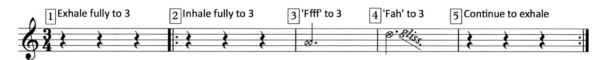

Try this cycle:

1. Exhale fully
2. Inhale fully while the Facilitator counts to 3
3. Exhale on a barely audible 'Ffff" while the Facilitator counts to 3
4. Move from 'Ffff' to 'Fah' on a higher tone, sliding down to a lower tone on continued exhalation
5. Complete the cycle by blowing out any remaining breath
6. As with the breathing cycle, lengthen the 'Fff' count over time

Hah!

Encourages diaphragmatic awareness and control.

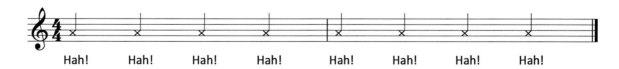

1. Place hands beneath rib cage across abdomen
2. Start with a sharp cough to feel muscles at work
3. Progress to 'Hah!' – encourage a short, sharp, non-breathy sound supported by abdominal muscles and diaphragm, not from the throat
4. Change sounds to other consonants: Dah! Kah! Pah! Gah! etc.

Tip: a policeman's 'belly-laugh' usually achieves the correct sound

Glissando slides

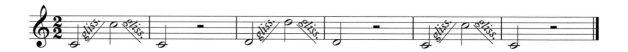

- Slide from note to note through the whole scale
- Use 'Nyah' or 'Mwah' to encourage an open vowel sound
- Notice the mid-scale voice break and change from chest to head voice
- Ensure mouth relaxed and well opened; support the high and low notes equally

Feeling catty?

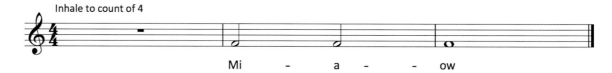

1. Inhale to count of 4
2. Exhale on 'Mi' – through to 'ah' and finish on 'ow' articulating through each vowel sound
3. Keep the sound bright – imagine an Italian, aristocratic cat
4. Ensure a forward-moving sound; do not allow the 'ow' to retreat to the back of the throat
5. Repeat on an ascending and descending scale, keeping a smooth, controlled sound

Alleluia

NOTE: boxed numbers indicate entry points for singing in rounds

Arr. Sonia Page

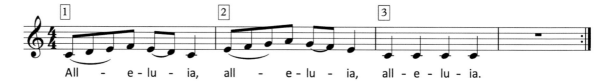

This effective warm-up is so simple yet incredibly flexible.

Consider:

- A soft 'Ah' on 'Alleluia' starting with an open, relaxed mouth
- Work through each vowel keeping a forward sound
- Smile: it's supposed to sound happy even if sung gently!
- Effective dynamics are achieved by growing louder then softer within each 'Alleluia'

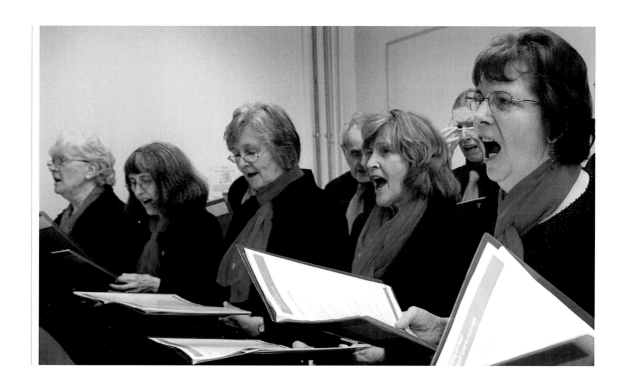

Belle mama

Trad.

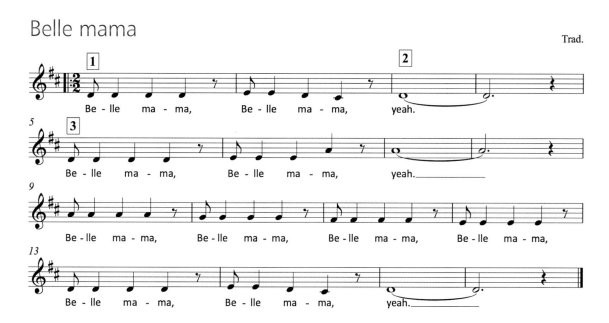

Belle mama delivers instant musical pleasure with its beautiful harmonies and African pulse. It provides a workout for facial and respiratory muscles as well as the brain. Consider the following:

- Tempo: a slow or lively tempo works equally well and provides variety

- Articulation: ensure a firm 'B' on Belle and 'M' on Mama throughout

- Breath control: hold 'yeah' for the full count while supporting the exhalation, then snatch a full breath ready for the next phrase. Ensure jaw is loose and mouth open for a full vowel sound

- Smile: this song demands a relaxed, happy and lively disposition

- Parts: consider singing once in unison then several times in two or three parts (see numbered entry points)

Tip: this is a fantastic icebreaker when groups come together, and lends itself to audience participation.

Senwa dedende

Trad. African

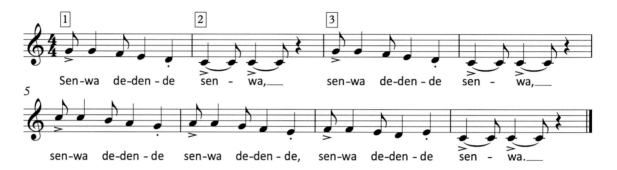

Sen-wa de-den - de sen - wa,___ sen-wa de-den - de sen - wa,___

sen-wa de-den - de sen-wa de-den - de, sen-wa de-den - de sen - wa.___

This beautiful song is one component of a longer Ghanaian narrative, which tells the story of a lazy vulture who has forgotten where he has built his nest.

- Encourage definite, confident consonants to enhance rhythmic structure

- Consider the tempo; this song is effective at a variety of tempi and can be used by the facilitator to influence the mood or pace of the session

- Suggest the group walks around the room while singing (if able); when sung as a round the combination of movement with harmonic structure promotes a relaxed yet purposeful atmosphere

- Accompany with drums, shakers etc. to add to the ambience

- Imagine an African tone and feel to the sound

Tip: this song can be used to promote unity and a sense of welcome within the group by encouraging eye contact and opening arms to one another in a gesture of greeting at the start of each phrase. Give it a try and watch the expression on the singers' faces.*

*Thanks to Jonathan Barnes of Canterbury Christ Church University for sharing this idea.

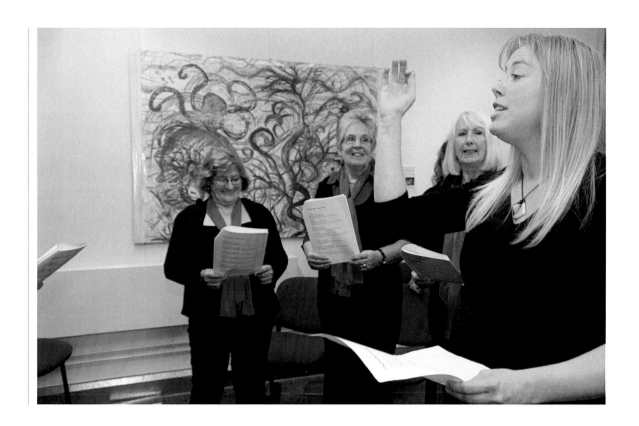

Conducting tips

Conducting, for the uninitiated, can be daunting. How does one demonstrate tempo, start the song, keep the group together and, crucially, finish at the same time? Every conductor's style is individual and necessarily so, for one size does not fit all. This section aims to equip the novice choir leader with basic tips and suggestions. However, it is highly recommended that where possible peer review is actively sought and utilised. It is not essential that a formal conducting technique for time signatures is employed. A clear beat, however demonstrated, will suffice.

Do:

- Practise at home: make sure you know what your left and right arms are doing. If one seems to have a mind of its own, don't use it until it behaves. Small, controlled, consistent, single-fingered movements are more effective than wild, bilateral arm waving which changes style with each song. Decide how you will encourage the group to get louder and softer and be consistent.

- Stand still: Unless the group is moving around the room as part of the singing, it is strongly advised that you remain a static visual point of reference. Remember that some of your participants may have mobility difficulties that reduce head and neck movements. Some may also struggle with manipulating music, page turning and sitting or standing up. Standing still raises the likelihood of their undivided attention and greater responsiveness to your conducting. Resist the urge to lunge toward sections to bring them in – they will learn to watch you.

- Keep it simple: if you are new to conducting the following components should suffice and may be all you need for your particular group:

- Prior to singing (when the group is starting out) familiarise the group with your conducting methods for counting in and getting louder and softer

- Count a clear beat to set the tempo (speed) before singing starts

- Keep the beat clear throughout the song

- Clearly signal the final beat to finish the song

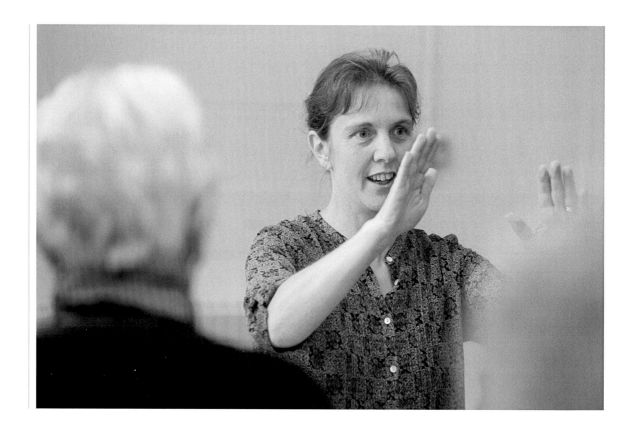

- Make eye contact: if you are buried in your music or word sheet you will not see how your group is singing. Familiarise yourself with the songs so that you spend more time looking at the singers than at your copy. They need to see your face as well as your arms and hands.

Don't:

- Panic if you get it wrong. That's 'don't panic'. You will almost certainly start a song at the wrong tempo and pitch at some point. Be prepared to laugh, raise your eyes heavenward and start again. Your group will love you more if you can see the funny side of things.

- Hide behind a music stand. Try to ensure your upper body and face is visible to all. You may need to stand on a stage block or step - anything to ensure everyone can see you.

Tip: conducting starts with your facial features and ends with your arm movements. Signal your intention with eye contact, smiles, nods etc. Don't worry if you feel out of your depth to start with; you will develop your own style and grow in confidence, and your group will respond to you accordingly.

Peer review can be a very positive experience. Choose someone you trust – preferably a more experienced choir leader or musician who will be honest with you. Ask them to assess whether your direction was clear and to suggest ways to enhance your technique.

Observe and experience other choir leaders' conducting. If possible, attend another singing group session as a participant and reflect on the conducting and leadership style employed by the facilitator. Ask yourself whether you felt adequately directed, encouraged and informed and how that experience might influence your own style.

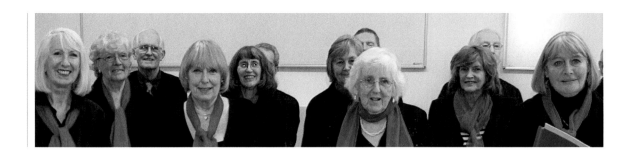

Repertoire

Singing is a joy, but choosing a repertoire may not always feel quite so joyful at times. Sometimes a particular song stands out as a 'must-do', yet at other times you may find yourself searching for inspiration. The following tips and examples may assist, but you should feel confident in choosing different material. Particular songs may suit one group but be rejected by another. Some of the singing for health groups utilising the following repertoire have included songs reflecting their multicultural membership.

Your choice of repertoire should reflect your confidence and ability as a facilitator. If you are musically competent and able to arrange harmony, teach individual parts and supply an accompaniment then you have an advantage, but none of these skills is absolutely necessary. Your group will gain great pleasure from singing even if all they have is a word-sheet and a pitch pipe for the starting note.

Tip: start with material that you know or can learn quickly yourself. You need to know a song before you can teach or lead it.

It is useful to have songs that vary in length, style, speed, difficulty and familiarity. Consider the health problems affecting your members and try to accommodate where possible. For example, if your singers have breathing difficulties they may find it discouraging to be asked to tackle songs requiring long, slow phrasing. Similarly, a group beset by terminal illness or bereavement may find it difficult to sing highly emotive material. Your group will, in time, express a preference for certain styles and you may decide that their dynamic suits a particular type of song, but do not allow this to become too restrictive. A varied repertoire should bring pleasure to all - including you. Please use the following examples as a catalyst for your own choices and direction.

Warm-up songs to get things going

- Belle Mama
- Senwa Dedende
- Lou Lou Medley
- Alleluia

Songs with short phrases

- Rhythm and Syncopation
- Shalom
- My Hat
- Quartermaster's Store
- Singing in the Rain
- My Bonnie Lies Over the Ocean

Songs with longer phrases

- Edelweiss
- Somewhere Over the Rainbow
- Moon River
- Skye Boat Song
- Waltzing Matilda

Copyright Issues

Please familiarise yourself with issues of copyright. It is an offense to copy or reproduce words or music without the permission of the composer/author. Help and advice regarding copyright is widely available on the Internet. You may find the following websites useful:

www.prsformusic.com

www.copyrightservice.co.uk

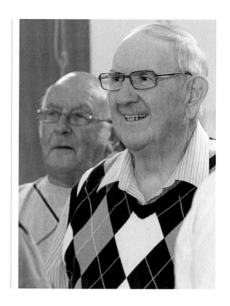

Session Example

Timing (approximate)	Activity	Rationale
5 minutes	Welcome – especially to any new members; brief outline of the session	New members may feel nervous and intimidated by the challenge ahead
10 minutes	Physical and vocal warm-ups: • Posture • Breathing • Vocal exercises	Prepares body and mind to sing; encourages relaxation and wellbeing
20 minutes	Sing 2-3 short songs Learn a new song or work in more detail on something fairly new	Shorter phrases or short songs provide a quick route to singing success which boost confidence and encourages relaxation
5 minutes	Revisit: Posture Breathing Cycle	Discourages poor posture and reminds the group of the importance of employing breathing techniques whilst singing; provides a short respite
15 minutes	Sing longer or more challenging songs. Explore new or difficult material Practise harmonies etc.	Now well warmed-up, the group may be able to tackle longer phrases or songs with a wider range
5 minutes	Close the session with discussion of what has been learned and achieved	Focuses minds on what has been achieved

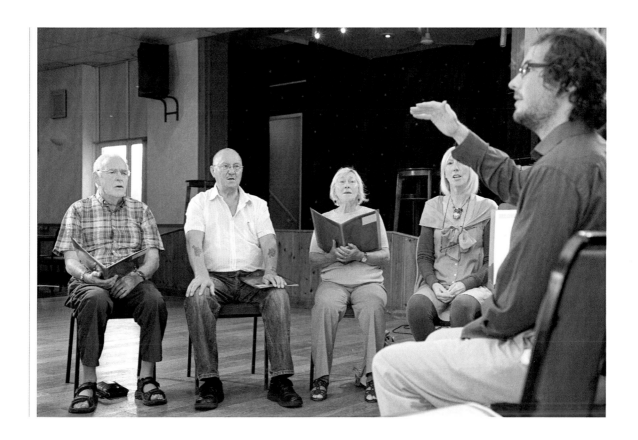

Getting Started

Still interested and keen to embark on a worthwhile, exciting venture? Your thoughts may now be drawn to the practicalities of getting your group started, which can be as simple as meeting in your front room with a few folks to enjoy a sing-along. However, with a little more planning and a structured approach, a new group can successfully find its feet from day one and adapt en route as required.

Who?

You may naturally assume that you'll run the group, and that may well be the case initially. However, for your protection and sanity it would be advisable to assemble a small committee, or at the very least two people to take on the role of Treasurer. Relinquishing some organisational responsibility enables you to focus on musical provision, which is liberating.

When?

Session timings often depend upon availability of a suitable venue, but experience suggests that early afternoon (2-3pm) is popular with many older people, and Saturday morning also works for many. It may be useful to plan sessions for term-time only as venues such as churches or village halls are often booked up for holiday events (clubs, drama productions etc.) In addition, you and they may well appreciate a break during school holidays.

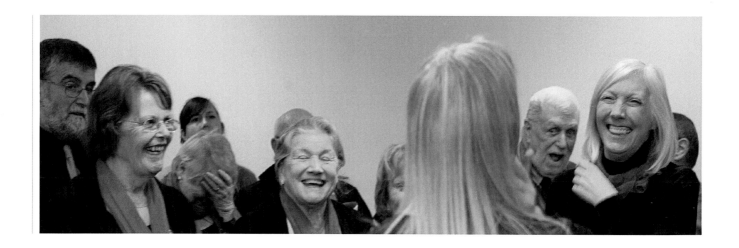

Where?

Choice of venue is vitally important and can encourage or deter attendance. Wherever you meet, consider the following factors:

- Heating: is the venue adequately heated and ventilated?
- Access: can participants reach the venue by public transport?
- Parking: essential when transporting equipment such as a keyboard or refreshments, and to those for whom public transport is not an option.
- Cost: sometimes the cheapest option is not the most suitable.
- Facilities: toilets, tea/coffee facilities, disabled access.

Tip: engagement with the hall manager and gaining his or her cooperation is invaluable.

Advertising

- Flyers can be made on home computers and given to surgeries, shops, cafés, social groups, libraries, supermarkets, dentists, vets, churches, sheltered housing etc.
- Local newspapers: there may be a charge involved but worth taking out a small advert and inviting local press to an event.
- Give flyers to your group members to use as personal invitations.

Money matters

- As previously mentioned, it is good practice to have two nominated Treasurers.
- Your fees: be careful not to under-price yourself. Find out what other facilitators charge and ensure you are paid fairly. Remember that you will be spending several hours each week preparing material as well as delivering the sessions.
- Subs: groups are commonly funded through membership subscription and the amount varies according to requirements. Consider your costs (venue, fees, insurance, photocopying) and ensure subs are sufficient to cover these. As your membership increases you may be able to reduce the amount.
- Funding: opportunities abound for funding applications, for example, town councils usually have an application process for non-profit groups; supermarkets often promote and encourage donations to local community schemes; performances provide opportunity for bucket-by-the-door donations and, once established, you may be able to apply for lottery funding. Donations via a 'bucket' collection for performances for local groups (e.g. Rotary clubs, churches) raise funds and such events are fun as well as invaluable for raising the group's profile.

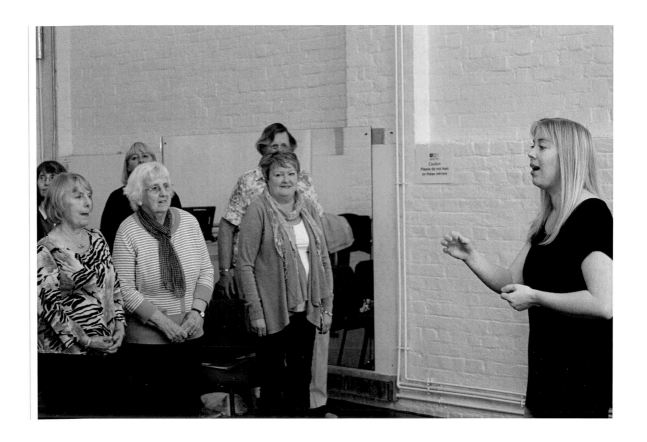

Insurance

- Consider personal insurance for public liability cover as well as other benefits including instrument damage protection.

- Check that your venue has insurance including public liability.

- Your choir may wish to take out its own insurance, which is usually not expensive and will ensure it is covered to perform anywhere.

Tip: the Musicians' Union and Making Music both offer excellent advice regarding the practicalities of running a choir including insurance, writing constitutions and performers' rights.

And finally

Singing is good for you. Not only will you be providing a fun, beneficial, life-affirming experience for your participants, you will find that the process of facilitation brings reward. You will discover that your efforts positively affect the lives of ordinary people even when you think you have not performed particularly well. Occasionally you will feel as though you are making no progress and that musically there are mountains to climb, but then a member will tell you what a particular song means to them, how much they enjoyed the singing today and what a lifeline it is for them. Then you will go home knowing that your efforts are worthwhile and that many of those for whom you have just provided an hour's enjoyment, social fulfilment and health-promoting exercise are counting the minutes until the next session.

In association with:

"These will be invaluable texts for anyone interested in music, health and wellbeing. Not only are they concise, clear and accessible but they provide exemplary examples of much needed research exploring the benefits of musical participation."

Professor Raymond MacDonald,
University of Edinburgh

"The Sidney de Haan Centre is to be congratulated for their work in first obtaining strong evidence for the benefits of singing and then creating these pamphlets so as to translate findings into community practice. The well organized presentation serves as a model for other countries and deserves recognition for showing the way to more initiatives both within and beyond the UK."

Professor Annabel J. Cohen, Director, AIRS
(Advancing Interdisciplinary Research in Singing)
University of Prince Edward Island, Canada

"Clear, concise and thoughtful guides that will help community musicians understand health issues and healthcare systems; and health professionals understand the role of good-quality singing work in a range of conditions."

Kathryn Deane,
Director, Sound Sense

"I cannot praise these Guide packs highly enough. I have been running training courses for those wishing to run groups and choirs since 1988. Increasingly people coming for training wish to work in the area of singing for health and well being, many of them bringing relevant backgrounds in the health and caring professions. The practical suggestions lay out all the essential aspects of running non-judgmental and inclusive groups."

Frankie Armstrong, Founder,
The Natural Voice Practitioners' Network

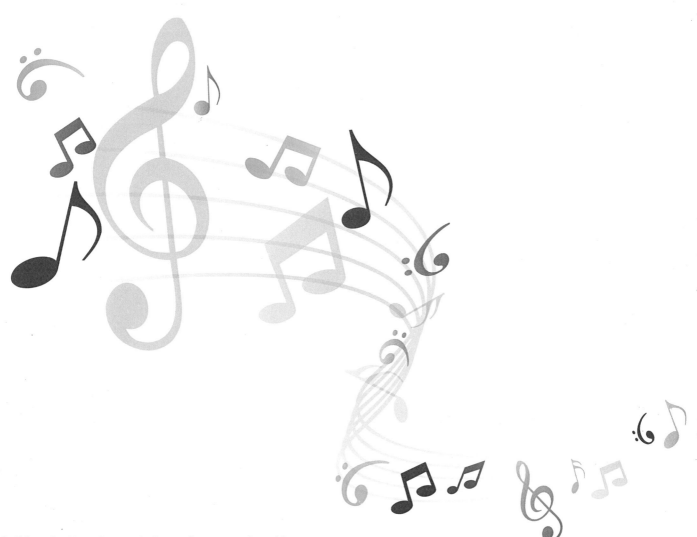

Canterbury Christ Church University, 65-69 The Block,
Tontine Street, Folkestone, Kent, England, CT20 1JR
Telephone: 01303 220 870

www.canterbury.ac.uk/research/centres/SDHR